I GOT DA SUGA BUT DA SUGA AIN'T GOT ME

THE MUST-HAVE GUIDE TO DEALING WITH DIABETES AND FINDING HOPE AND HAPPINESS

DEANNA M. RICE, RN, BBA, MBA

ISBN: 978-1-943258-78-9
ISBN: 978-0-692-38364-4 (first printing)

Edited by: Elizabeth Russell

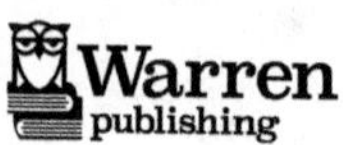

Published by Warren Publishing
Charlotte, NC
www.warrenpublishing.net
Printed in the United States

This book is dedicated to my beautiful daughters
Amaris, Constance, Brittany, Ashley, & Alexis.
Also to all those who prayed and chanted
"Grow Nori Grow." To my granddaughter, Nori Blu,
the little light that brightened the world!

I would like to thank the following people
for their rock of support:
My Mommy (1)–Gloria Rookard
My Mommy (2)–Nita Williams
Sylky "Smooth" Johnson
Howard Rookard
Yo Erv McKoy
Da Suga Crew
Derek Gelispie
Jay Johnson, Jr.
Charlie Singfield

I would also like to give a special thanks to all those individuals who have given, loved, and supported this wonderful journey of healing through love. Thank you!

In loving memory of:

Claude Shuler
Maurine (Lucy) Shuler
Howard J. Rookard, Sr.
Derrick A. Rookard
Douglas S. Rookard, Jr.
Diane Munnerlyn-Jones
Arnold R. Pinkney
Baby L. J.

FOREWORD

Let's keep it simple, as a diabetic, I've found that diabetes is a daunting disease that can very easily take control and devastate those in its path. Being able to understand and manage "da suga" is paramount to living a long and healthy life with diabetes. This book is a must-read for the entire family.

Dr. George C. Fraser
Frasernet.com

Diabetes is a formidable, relentless, incurable disease. It has been studied, written about, and researched. It causes physical, mental, and emotional trauma in its victims, which in its wake, leaves devastation and even death. This edition attempts to educate and motivate. It comes from the pen of a nurse who has experienced many stages of diabetic trauma over the years. Some patients could manage their disease process while others were negligent, non-compliant, or just plain in denial until devastation took over. Thus, *I Got Da Suga* was born.

Gloria S. Rookard, CEO, RN, PNP

INTRODUCTION

I'm at work and it's my turn to admit the next new patient to the floor. This patient happens to be an elderly African American male about 5'10" tall, with an unkempt salt and pepper afro; big working hands; one beat up, low-top Converse on his left foot; and a wash cloth and plastic bag rubber banded around the right foot. He is fifty-three and looks seventy.

While talking to this gentleman, I learn that about two weeks ago he was walking in the house barefoot and stepped on a tack. He didn't think about it much because it didn't bother him. He never noticed the wound was getting worse because he didn't look at his foot. He stated his legs and feet are usually tingly and numb. As time progressed, his wife noticed a foul odor under the covers when they got in and out of bed. When she looked at the bottom of his foot, there was a sore between the big toe and the second toe on the right. It was draining some pus-like fluid and the odor was unbearable. His wife suggested a ride to the hospital, and that is when they decided to wrap his foot in a washcloth and a plastic bag.

One of my first questions to the patient was, "Do you have diabetes?" His answer was, "I don't know nuthin' about no diabetes, but I know I got da suga."

"The sugar?" I said.

"Yes," he replied. "That's what my grandmother used to say when you had too much sugar in your blood."

"Well sir, I'm afraid it is a little more complicated than that. We will get you some information that will help you understand your diabetes and possibly safeguard you against this happening again."

Although the odor was apparent once I entered his room, it was overwhelming when the plastic bag was removed from his foot. If you have ever smelled rotting flesh, it is a smell not forgotten. When I examined his toe with the doctor, I knew there was a strong possibility he would leave the hospital without his toe, or possibly his whole foot, and I was right. Fortunately, it was only his toe.

This story, although details may differ, is prevalent among diabetic patients, especially African American males. It has often been said that diabetes is a relentless disease. Its process is slow, meticulous, and can be gruesome. There are no spared organs (eyes, heart, kidneys, etc.). It slowly claims pieces of your body one at a time, toe by toe, foot by foot, and limb by limb.

In 2010, there were 73,000 non-traumatic amputations performed on adults aged twenty and older and sixty percent of those amputations were on people with diagnosed diabetes. It has earned its place as the seventh leading cause of death in the United States, singlehandedly killing more Americans each year than breast cancer and AIDS combined.

Currently, 30.3 million people or 9.4 percent of the population are diagnosed with diabetes, and there are an estimated 7.2 million more people who don't know they have the disease, or "da suga," as it is often called by older African Americans.

This introduction is not meant to scare you, but to make you aware of the seriousness of this disease, how it affects your body, and how to safeguard yourself from its complications. Now, there is good news and bad news. The bad news is there is no cure for diabetes. The good news is it's a progressive disorder that can be managed through diet, exercise, and proper monitoring. In the pages ahead, we will discuss some common diabetic myths, facts, and stats, testing and diagnosis, signs and symptoms, complications, "Da Suga" basics, and "Da Suga" Survival Kit.

Welcome to *I Got Da Suga ... But Da Suga Ain't Got Me.*

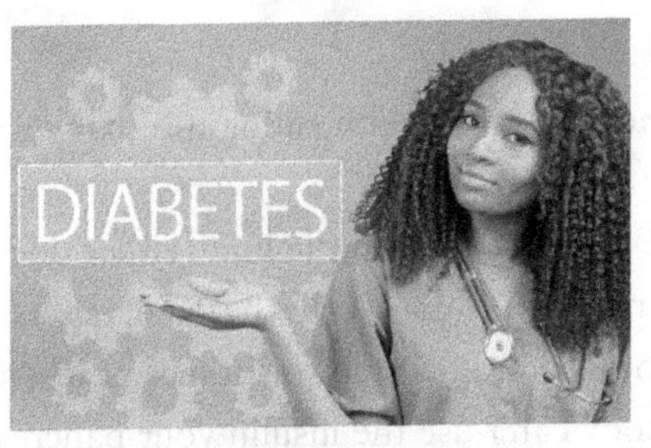

"DA SUGA" MYTHS, FACTS, AND STATS

There are many myths about "da suga" that show how much work still needs to be done to educate the public about the seriousness and devastating effects of diabetes. These myths continue to resonate and live on among the general population. They are passed from generation to generation.

MYTH 1: DIABETES IS *CAUSED* BY EATING TOO MUCH SUGAR.

Fact: There are different types of diabetes, but for the purpose of exposing this as myth, let's look at Type 1 and Type 2 diabetes.

Type 1 diabetes is caused by genetics and other unknown factors. Type 1 diabetes is when your body makes no insulin. Insulin is made in your pancreas by beta cells. When you have Type 1 diabetes, these cells have been destroyed. This type of diabetes is usually discovered in children and young adults. Only five percent of all diabetics have this type of diabetes, and this has nothing to do with eating too many candy bars or sugary drinks.

Type 2 diabetes is when the body either doesn't make enough insulin, or your cells become resistant to the insulin you produce. Insulin resistance is when the cells in your body can't use the insulin your pancreas makes, even though it is working efficiently. When your cells are resistant, they can't get "da suga" into the cells for energy. This is also not caused by the amount of sugar you consume, but by your body's reaction between your cells and the insulin you make.

Myth 2: Diabetes is not a serious disease.

Fact: This has to be one of the most dangerous myths. Diabetes has been connected to several other serious illnesses, including heart disease and stroke. Two out of three people with diabetes die from one of these two illnesses. There are many other complications associated with diabetes, such as damage to the eyes, feet, and skin, as well as kidney disease and neuropathy, which is nerve damage to the feet that causes numbness. All these complications make diabetes very serious.

Myth 3: If you are overweight, you will develop Type 2 diabetes.

Fact: Weight is considered a risk factor for diabetes. A "risk factor" is something that increases a person's chance of developing a particular disease. It is not a cause of "Da Suga." Below you will find several risk factors for developing diabetes, none of which are causes. The risk factors are as follows:

- ❑ Forty-five years of age or older
- ❑ Heredity
- ❑ Race (African American, Hispanic/Latino, American Indian, Pacific Islander, or Asian American)
- ❑ High cholesterol
- ❑ Inactivity
- ❑ Diabetes while pregnant (gestational diabetes)

We have no control over some of the risk factors, such as age, heredity, and race, but we can control our diets and exercise routines to reduce our risks of developing diabetes.

Myth 4: You can catch diabetes from someone else.

Fact: Catching "da suga" this way is impossible. It is not like the chickenpox or a cold. The disease is not passed on through direct or indirect contact, airborne droplets, or germs on surfaces. This disease is something researchers have found you are predisposed to inherit. You can also develop "da suga" by not effectively managing the many risk factors associated with the disease, such as high blood pressure or inactivity.

Myth 5: All diabetics must have insulin.

Fact: Not all diabetics use insulin to control their disease. There are many diabetics whose diabetes is managed through exercise and proper nutrition. There are others who are able to manage their diabetes through oral medications or a combination of the above. The only diabetics who must have insulin are those with Type 1 diabetes. All Type 1 diabetics need insulin to manage "da suga," whereas Type 2 diabetics may or may not need insulin. Remember, a Type 1 diabetic's body does not make any insulin, so it is a must for them.

Myth 6: Diabetic patients are more susceptible to colds and illnesses in general.

Fact: This is not true. A person with diabetes that is managed well is no more likely to become sick with a cold or illness than anyone else. However, when a diabetic does become ill, their diabetes becomes harder to control, so their risk of complications is greater.

Myth 7: I have to take insulin, so my diabetes is severe.

Fact: Insulin is only prescribed for Type 2 diabetics when diet alone or diet along with oral or non-insulin injectable diabetes drugs do not provide enough control. Insulin is simply a means of helping "da suga" get into the cells. It is not an indicator of the severity of your condition. Remember, your body makes insulin naturally to assist the cells in getting the glucose to use for energy.

Myth 8: High blood sugar levels are fine for some, while for others they are a sign of diabetes.

Fact: High blood sugar levels are never normal for anyone. Some illnesses, mental stress, and steroids can cause temporary spikes in "da suga" levels in people without diabetes. If your blood sugar levels are higher than normal or you have sugar in your urine, you should be checked for diabetes.

Myth 9: I know when my blood sugar levels are high or low.

Fact: Very high or very low blood sugar may cause various symptoms such as weakness, fatigue, and extreme thirst. However, blood sugar levels need to be fluctuating drastically for symptoms to be felt. Never guess about your sugar levels. Patients who think their sugar is high or low based on how they feel will often find after checking that they were wrong. The only way to really tell is by checking.

Myth 10: Children can outgrow diabetes.

Fact: Nearly all children with diabetes have Type 1. This is where insulin-making beta cells in the pancreas have been destroyed. These cells never come back. This is the primary reason people with Type 1 diabetes will always need insulin. Let us not forget that there is no cure for diabetes, so it is impossible to outgrow "da suga." It can only be managed.

A startling truth about "da suga" is that as of 2015, 30.3 million Americans or 9.4% of the population have diabetes, and there has been a steady growth since 2012. According to the latest statistics from the American Diabetes Association, every twenty-one seconds someone is diagnosed with diabetes. In 2015, over 322 billion dollars were spent treating diabetes. This is up from 2012 where 176 billion dollars were spent in direct medical costs such as doctor visits and hospital stays, plus sixty-nine billion dollars were spent in reduced productivity or sick days. A diabetic's health care cost is two and a half times higher than a non-diabetic's.

Approximately 79,535 death certificates listed diabetes as an underlying cause in 2015 with a total of 252,806 death certificates listing diabetes as a contributing factor.

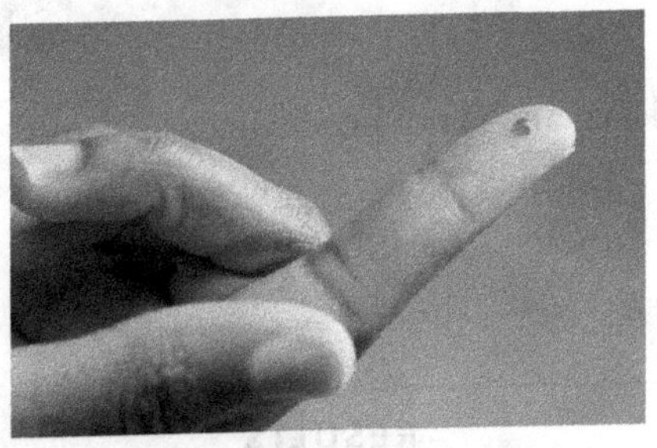

WHAT IS "DA SUGA?"

"Da suga" (diabetes) is classified as a metabolism disorder. Metabolism is the way our bodies use digested food for energy and growth. Most of what we eat is broken down into glucose, which is the main source of fuel for our bodies.

Diabetes describes a group of metabolic diseases in which a person has high blood glucose either because insulin production is inadequate or non-existent, or the body's cells do not respond properly to insulin. A person with diabetes has a condition in which the quantity of glucose in the blood is too high. It's like a car with sugar in the gas tank. That car will run sluggishly unless the gas is cleaned and "da suga" is eliminated. "Da suga" doesn't dissolve in the tank, just as it doesn't dissolve in your blood without treatment.

There is such a thing as pre-diabetes, or you *almost* got "da suga." This is where your blood glucose levels are higher than normal but not high enough to classify you as diabetic. In this instance, the cells in your body are becoming resistant to insulin or your pancreas is wearing down and is not producing an adequate amount of insulin. "Da suga" chart below shows blood sugar test results and the classification of your diabetes based on the results:

RESULTS	
Normal	Between 70 mg/dl–100 mg/dl
Pre-diabetes	101 mg/dl–125 mg/dl
Diabetes	Greater than 126 mg/dl

There are four methods of testing and subsequently diagnosing diabetes:

1. A1C test;
2. Fasting Plasma Glucose (FPG);
3. Oral Glucose Tolerance Test (OGTT);
4. The Random Plasma Glucose test.

A diagnosis is generally made after two or more elevated results, except during the A1C test and the Random Plasma Glucose test. The testing is not complicated, but is required in order to accurately make "da suga" diagnosis.

First, let's look at the A1C or Glycated Hemoglobin test. This test measures the amount of hemoglobin, which is protein, found in red blood cells. Red blood cells carry oxygen from the lungs to all cells in the body. They also pick up glucose in the bloodstream along the way. The A1C test measures the average blood glucose and your body's management of this glucose over the past three months. So, how is that? Blood glucose can be measured this way because the red blood cells in your body live for about 120 days and are continuously replaced with new cells. Since the cells live for so many days, it allows us to look at how well your body manages "da suga" over a three-month period. For example, if you get your A1C test taken in March, it measures the amount of glucose that is broken down and connected to your hemoglobin in December, January, and February. Remember, hemoglobin travels through your body delivering oxygen, nutrients, and glucose for use. The reason this is a three-month measurement is because once your glucose hooks up with your hemoglobin, it's for life. Divorce rate with these cells is 0%. Only 5% of your hemoglobin should be used this way. The more glucose in your blood, the higher the percentage of hemoglobin that gets the hook up. If you don't have diabetes, only 5% of all hemoglobin is broken down or hooked up with glucose. If you have diabetes, that number is higher, usually greater than 6.5%. This number can fluctuate from time to time based on how well you manage "da suga."

A1C TEST	RANGE
Normal	Less than 5.7%
Pre-Diabetes	Between 5.7% - 6.4%
Diabetes	Greater than 6.5%

Check with your health care professional to see how often you should have this measured, but the recommendation is at least twice a year.

Next let's look at the fasting Plasma Glucose test. This test measures your blood sugar level after not eating or drinking for at least eight hours. Water is permitted. The blood sample needs to be taken before any insulin or oral anti-diabetic medications have been taken. This test is usually conducted in the morning before breakfast. A diabetic diagnosis is made when two separate results are greater than 126 mg/dl. This test is the preferred method of diagnosis.

FASTING PLASMA GLUCOSE TEST	RANGE
Normal	Less than 100 mg/dl
Pre-diabetes	Between 100 mg/dl–125 mg/dl
Diabetes	Greater than 126 mg/dl

The OGTT or Oral Glucose Tolerance test checks your blood glucose in the morning after a ten- to twelve- hour fast. A fasting blood sample is obtained. Then you will be asked to drink a special sweet-flavored beverage and within five minutes after drinking the beverage, the first blood glucose sample is obtained. More blood samples are taken every thirty minutes for two hours. You will not be able to eat, drink, or smoke during this test. This test measures how the body processes glucose. This is the most sensitive test for the diagnosis of diabetes. Two or more elevated levels during this test are an indicator of diabetes.

OGTT	RANGE
Normal	Less than 140 mg/dl
Pre-diabetes	Between 140 mg/dl–199 mg/dl
Diabetes	Greater than 200 mg/dl

The Random Plasma Glucose test checks blood glucose any time of the day. A result of greater than 200 mg/dl would be considered diabetes.

It is important to be tested for diabetes if there is a chance you have "da suga" based on family history, age, or any other risk factors previously listed.

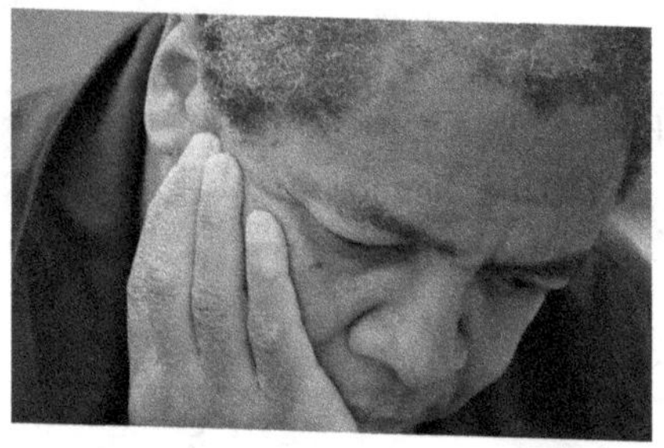

"DA SUGA" SIGNS AND SYMPTOMS

There are different signs and symptoms depending on whether "da suga" is high (hyperglycemia) or low (hypoglycemia), and certain things that can be done to safeguard against a low blood sugar or high blood sugar attack.

Let's first take a look at low blood sugar, which is a blood sugar result below 70 mg/dl. When your blood sugar is low, you will experience cool, clammy skin. You will begin to perspire profusely and become anxious, nervous, shaky, or irritable. It may even become serious enough for you to experience mental confusion or slip into a coma. You will become unusually weak and may have double or blurred vision, increased hunger, and rapid heartbeat or palpitations.

There are four common causes of low blood sugar and they are as follows:

1. Too much insulin;
2. Exercise;

3. Not enough food; and/or
4. Alcohol consumption.

It is wise to educate your family on these symptoms so they are able to recognize when your blood sugar is low and can assist you in returning your blood sugar to safe levels with proper treatment. Usually treatment for a mild low blood sugar attack would include the consumption of between 10 grams and 15 grams of carbohydrates, which could be one or more of the following:

- Glucose tablets or glucose gel
- ½ cup of fruit juice
- ½ cup of regular (non-diet) soft drink
- 8 oz. of skim milk
- 6–10 pieces of hard candy
- 4 cubes of sugar
- 6 saltines
- 3 graham crackers
- 1 tablespoon of honey or syrup

Once one of these has been administered, the blood glucose test should be repeated in fifteen minutes. Treat and check "da suga" every fifteen minutes until the symptoms resolve and blood sugar levels are returned to a safe range. Repeat treatment if symptoms do not resolve and blood sugar levels remain under 70 mg/dl. If your next meal is more than an hour away, you should eat a small snack rich in carbohydrates and protein. If this does not work and your symptoms become worse, you should seek medical attention right away.

Be aware of how you're feeling because the onset of low blood sugar may be subtle. It may be caused by a combination of things such as other medications (including certain types of blood pressure medications), a fall in hormone levels, or something as simple as switching to a new bottle of insulin. (A fresh bottle is more potent.) Remember, there does not have to be a direct cause to trigger your low blood sugar episode. It could be nothing more than the erratic absorption of insulin, which can happen to even careful diabetic patients.

For high blood sugar, the symptoms are different. You will be hot with dry skin, which can be a sign of dehydration. Your breathing will become rapid and deep, with a fruity odor in your breath. You may be alert but you could also become drowsy or stuporous, not stupid but lethargic or sleepy. You may also experience abdominal cramping, nausea and/or vomiting, and you may begin passing sugar particles in your urine.

High blood sugar can be more troublesome because of the process. When your blood sugar levels are high, the "Poly P Three" show up: Polyuria or frequent urination, polydipsia or excessive thirst, and polyphagia or intense hunger. These three are in direct relation to your blood sugar levels being high or your tank being full of "da suga" if you will. Your body is amazing. It is built to survive and protect itself from destruction, so it begins to signal your body to do something about the high concentration of "da suga" in the blood, thus Poly P Three.

Let's explore what happens when your blood sugar is high. You will notice that you become increasingly thirsty. This is your body's way of trying to dilute the sugar in your blood. You begin to drink a lot, noticing that your thirst is never quenched. The intense thirst leads to frequent urination. This is your kidneys taking action to help your body rid itself of the excessive amount of sugar in the blood stream. Your kidneys will begin to take water from your blood in order to dilute the glucose and, in turn, your bladder becomes full and you continue to urinate. Then, in the quest for more energy, you become hungry and you eat a lot, trying to replace the lost energy due to the sugar not making it into your cells.

When the Poly P Three are in full effect, the snowball begins. The frequent thirst leads to frequent urination, which leads to loss of electrolytes, which leads to dehydration. This then leads to a thicker blood concentration, decreased blood volume, and decreased circulation and poor tissue perfusion, especially to the brain. Then your body becomes acidic, leading to increased difficulty breathing. Your breath becomes fruity when the acetone is exhaled. Now you are in what we call a diabetic emergency based on the complications that have gone untreated. You should immediately seek medical attention!

Now, how high is "high?" A case in point is another patient I encountered during my nursing care. After being transferred to our floor from the Intensive Care Unit, we were aggressively monitoring this patient's blood sugar. I then reviewed his blood work and noticed that when he was admitted, his blood sugar had been at a whopping high 1493. Normal blood sugar is between 70 and 100. Amazed at the number and shocked that he was alive to talk about it, I asked him how in the world this could have happened. He stated that he had become very thirsty, and in an effort to quench his thirst he began drinking soda. He polished off two cases of soda before he had a convulsion, but then still drove himself to the hospital. During the course of all of this, he never checked his blood sugar. Now I don't recommend you try this at home. Luckily, his behavior did not have deadly consequences.

The following are complications of poorly controlled diabetes:

- **Eyes**—glaucoma, cataracts, diabetic retinopathy
- **Feet**—neuropathy, ulcers, gangrene, amputation
- **Skin**—infections and other skin disorders
- **Heart**—ischemic heart disease, diminished blood supply to the heart muscle
- **High Blood Pressure**—a common problem raising the risk of kidney disease, heart attack, or stroke
- **Mental Health**—depression, anxiety, and others
- **Hearing Loss**
- **Gum Disease**
- **Gastoparesis**—affecting stomach muscles causing them not to work properly

- **Ketoacidosis**—accumulation of ketones and acid in the blood
- **Neuropathy**—nerve damage, especially in the extremities
- **Nephropathy**—kidney disease
- **Peripheral Artery Disease**—may include tingling and pain in the legs or stroke
- **Erectile Dysfunction**
- **Infections**
- **Slow healing of wounds**

As you can see, the complications of diabetes are nothing to fool around with. It is vitally important to keep an eye on your sugar levels. You need to check often and treat as necessary.

"Don't let 'da suga' get you; you get 'da suga.'"

"DA SUGA" CHEAT SHEET

NORMAL BLOOD SUGAR 70–100 MG/DL

LOW BLOOD SUGAR: <70 MG/DL

Signs/symptoms

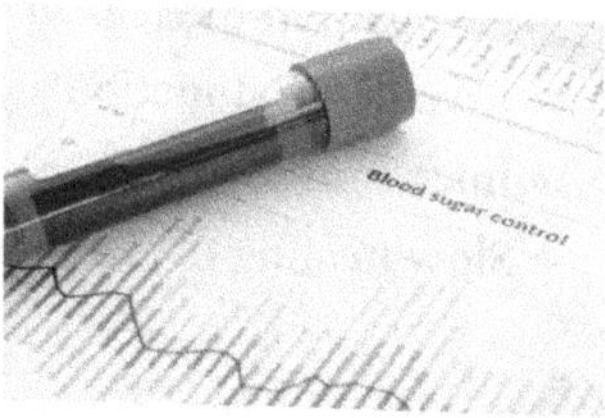

- Shakiness
- Nervousness/anxiety
- Clammy skin
- Sweating
- Confusion
- Irritability
- Rapid/fast heartbeat
- Hunger
- Light headedness/dizziness

Treatment

- 10–15 gm carbohydrates
- Recheck blood sugar every 15 minutes
- Eat small meal if next meal more than 1 hour away

HIGH BLOOD SUGAR: >126 MG/DL

Signs/symptoms

- Increased thirst
- Frequent urination
- Increased hunger
- Headaches
- Difficulty concentrating
- Blurred vision
- Weight loss

Treatment

- Insulin administration
- Call health care professional if BSG > 180 mg/dl

CURRENT MEDICATION LIST

Medication Name	Medication Dosage	How Many Times

Use this chart to always keep a current medication list handy. This way, in the event you have a diabetic episode, this information will be available.

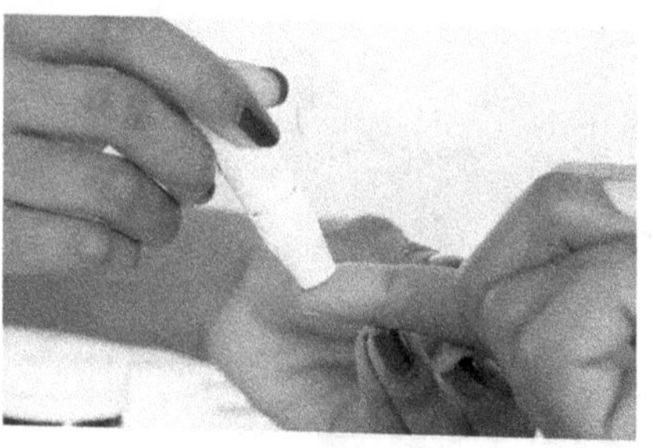

"DA SUGA" BASICS

When monitoring your blood sugar, it is important that you use the correct technique. This ensures proper monitoring and accurate treatment, if necessary, of any high or low result. There seems to be some controversy as to the reliability of "da suga" reading if you use the first drop of blood vs. the second drop of blood. Studies have shown that the reading can vary greatly based on the initial steps prior to the finger actually being pricked.

It is vitally important to start with clean, dry hands. If you can't start with clean, dry hands, then you should use the second drop of blood after wiping away the first drop with some clean, dry gauze or tissue. There is a sound medical reason why you should use the second drop of blood, not discussed here, but based on conducted studies. If the hands are washed and dried prior to self-monitoring, then it is okay to use the first drop of blood. This is only true after the hands have been washed and dried.

Steps to checking "da suga":

1. Wash and dry hands
2. Remove test strips
3. Insert test strips into the meter
4. Insert lancet into lancing device
5. Cock lancet
6. Choose puncture site
7. Wipe finger with alcohol swab
8. Dry finger with clean gauze or tissue
9. Prick finger
10. Place blood on test strip
11. Wait 15 seconds for result

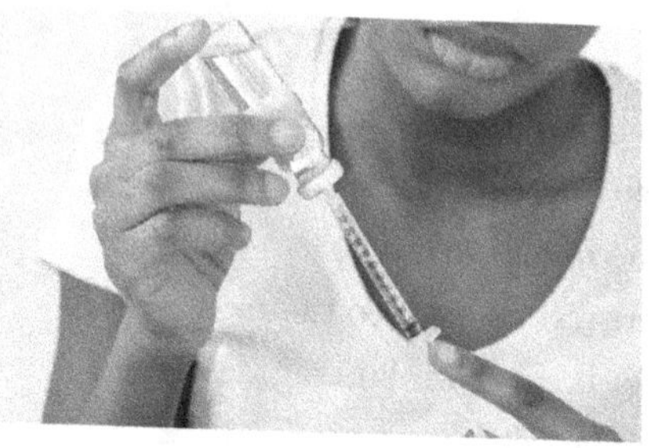

INSULIN

Insulin is a hormone secreted by beta cells in the pancreas that sends a signal to cells to start drawing nutrients from the blood. Without it, your cells would starve. Insulin also stimulates cells in the liver to restore glycogen and turns any excess sugar into fatty acids. This stops the body from breaking down fat in the tissue and using it for energy.

When you overdose on insulin, the insulin really lowers "da suga." Severe low blood sugar can cause the brain to shut down, resulting in a coma and/or death. Symptoms are mainly due to decreased brain activity and include fatigue, headache, confusion, hunger, and weakness.

There are many different types of insulin, which have different effects on how your body processes glucose. Your insulin regimen should be discussed with a medical professional to ensure maximum control. What is important is the fact that there are long-acting, intermediate-acting, short-acting, and fast-acting insulins. Long-acting insulin, such as Lantus, lasts for twenty four hours and begins working two to four hours after administration. This type covers you all day by releasing insulin little by little throughout the day to help you maintain your levels over a long period of time. An intermediate insulin such as the 70/30 mixture or NPH usually begins working in fifteen minutes and begins to peak or reach the height of its effectiveness between one and twelve hours. Depending on which insulin you are prescribed, some of the intermediate insulins also last twenty four hours.

The short-acting insulins begin working within thirty minutes and peak between two to twelve hours. When taking this type of insulin, you should eat within thirty minutes of insulin administration. The rapid-acting insulins such as Aspart or Lispro begin working within fifteen minutes of administration and usually peak within one to three hours and last up to five hours. These insulins should only be administered with food. This will avoid "da suga" dropping too fast.

A good rule of thumb when taking any insulin is to always remember to check "da suga" levels prior to administration and have a light snack or meal after the administration of any of the quicker acting insulins. Follow your health professional's diabetic plan for you and keep him or her informed of any changes you notice.

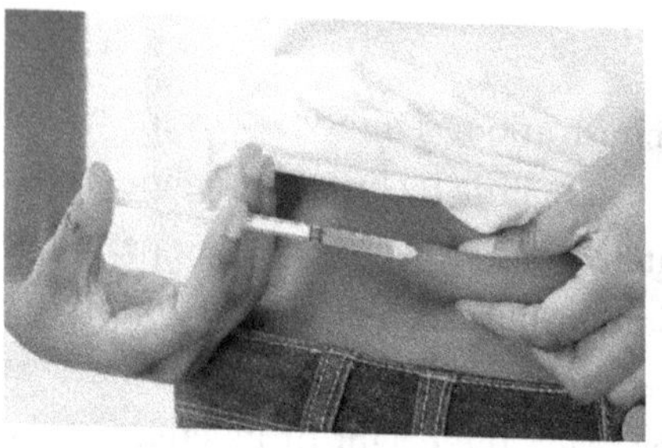

"DA SUGA" SITES

It is vitally important to rotate your injection sites when administering your insulin. Rotating where you give yourself insulin will decrease the risk of developing scar tissue, bumps, lumps, and dimpling under the skin. These bumps, lumps, and dimpling lead to slower absorption rates at these sites.

There are four recommended insulin injection sites and they are as follows:

1. The stomach
2. The buttocks
3. The outer thighs
4. The upper arms

(see diagram, pg. 32)

These places are recommended because they are the fattiest places on your body. Using these recommended locations will decrease your risk of possibly injecting the insulin into your muscle. Stay away from your belly button if your site of preference is the stomach. Also avoid the knee area and the muscular part of the upper arm. If you favor a particular part of your body for your injections, be sure to pick a location at least an inch away from the previous injection site so you are not weakening the fatty tissue under the skin and possibly causing nerve damage. If you notice over time that you are no longer able to feel the injections, this is a sign of damaged skin.

Remember: Rotate, rotate, rotate. Stick and move!

Stick Sites

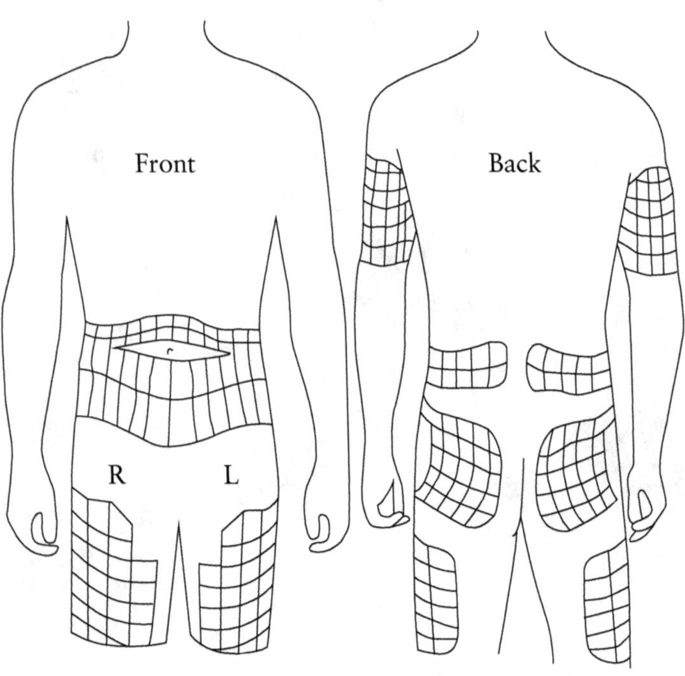

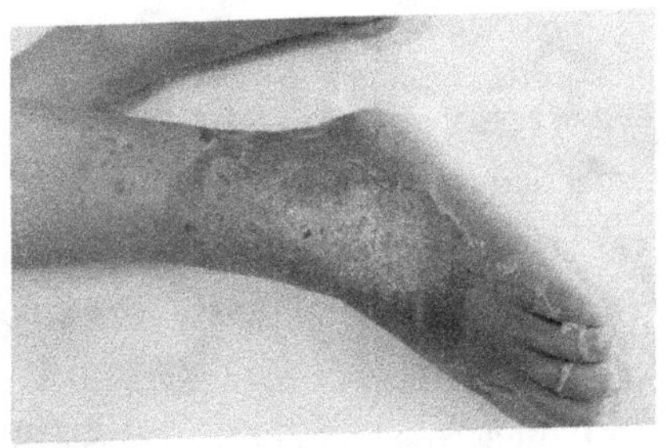

"DA SUGA" FOOT

You can't talk about "da suga" without talking about foot care and the importance of maintaining healthy feet and skin. Diabetics should have a system for continuously checking their feet and skin so they will not develop "da suga" foot. Please refer to the photos below to see pictures of what happens to diabetics and their feet if they don't keep them clean and dry or have proper management of "da suga."

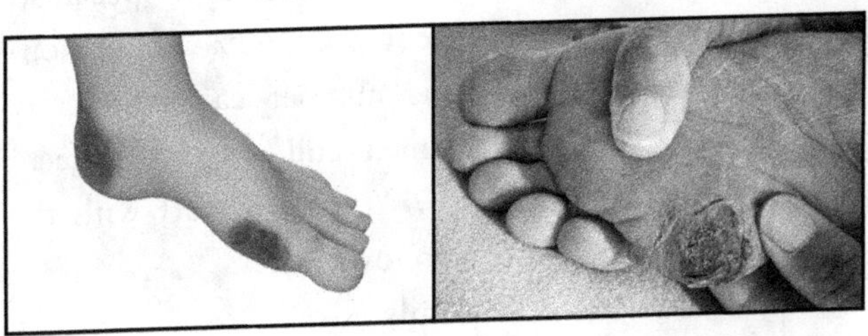

As you can see, the effects can be devastating. It used to be recommended that you not clip your toenails if you had diabetes. The recommendation was for you to see a podiatrist. Research has found that it is okay to manage your foot care, and clip your toenails, but they need to be clipped straight across and not too close to the skin. If you feel as though you are unable to manage this, then I encourage you to see a podiatrist and allow them to clip your nails or educate you on the proper technique.

I recommend that you check your feet often with a mirror or have someone else do the looking. Do your best to keep your feet clean and dry. Avoid walking around in your bare feet so you don't have an incident like my patient in the beginning of this booklet. Diabetic shoes are recommended and worn for the purpose of protecting and supporting the feet in order to prevent complications and the development of "da suga" foot. These shoes must be prescribed by your physician and properly fitted by a podiatrist or other foot specialist. As stated earlier, diabetics comprise 60% of all non-traumatic amputations. This number can be greatly reduced with proper management and care of your feet.

What is proper foot care? You must start with the basics and the basics are as follows:

- Clean and inspect feet daily
- Wear properly fitting shoes
- Avoid walking in bare feet
- Trim toenails properly

- Report non-healing breaks in the skin to your medical provider

As a diabetic, your risks are significantly higher for amputation. The most common reason for hospitalization among diabetics comes from foot injuries and poor skin management.

Remember to:

"Love a prick, save a limb.
Check 'da suga' often!"

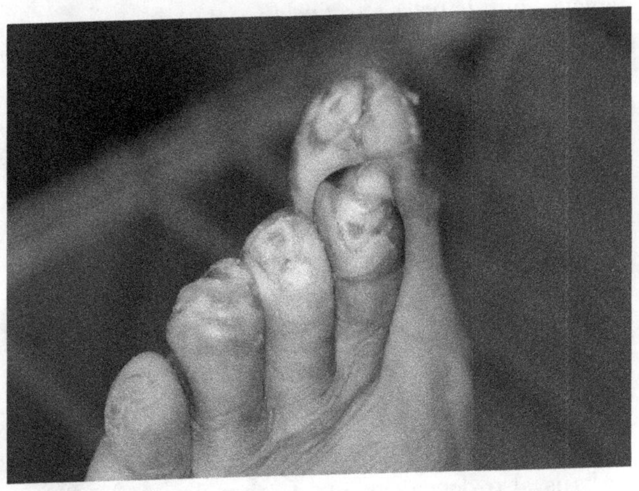

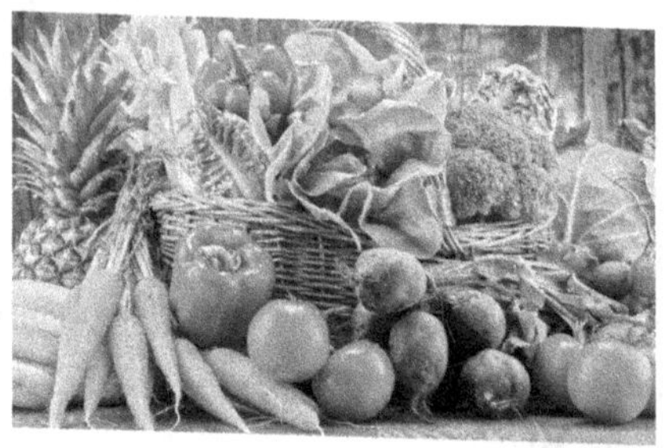

"DA SUGA" AND NUTRITION

You cannot educate anyone about diabetes without talking about nutrition and how it affects your blood sugar levels. Technically, there is no such a thing as a diabetic diet, but there are foods you should monitor and ways to balance your diet that will help you manage your diabetes effectively.

Food is made up of carbohydrates, protein, and fat. These are the components in food that affect "da suga." Out of the three of these, carbohydrates have the biggest effect on your blood glucose levels. Carbohydrates are usually found in starchy foods like rice, pasta, potatoes, and bread. The misunderstanding is that the best way to avoid carbohydrates is to simply remove them from your diet. This is not true. Carbohydrates (or carbs) are the main component that provide glucose for fuel, and it is recommended that diabetics receive half or more of their calories from carbs. Of course, the amount of carbs is also dependent upon other illnesses or issues complicating your diabetes. This is why education and nutritional counseling are important. There are many foods that are good for you that have carbohydrates in them. An example of these would be fruits, milk, yogurt, and smoothies. All of these foods are important for a healthy diet.

Protein is necessary in your diet for several reasons. One of the main functions of protein is to build lean muscle mass. It is an essential part of all diets. The good thing about protein and diabetes is that it does not contribute to spikes in your blood sugar levels. Protein is actually a good filler, slows the absorption of carbs, and allows you to eat less by keeping you full longer. Foods that are high in protein include cheese, meat, yogurt, beans, and nuts. When selecting meats, choose meats that are lean with little fat. This will help reduce your risk of high blood pressure and stroke.

Now let's talk about fat. There are good fats and bad fats, and just like protein and carbohydrates, you need some fat in your diet for vital organ function. There are different types of fats, for example, saturated and trans fats, monosaturated fats, and cholesterol. Now your objective is to try and avoid the bad fats, which are the saturated and trans fats, because they add to your risk of heart disease and stroke by adding plaque to your arteries. Monosaturated fats are considered the good fats and can help you get rid of cholesterol. Cholesterol is a fat-like substance that is already produced by your liver in a sufficient quantity, so limiting your cholesterol intake is important.

How do you know which fat is which? Well, here is some food for thought. The first thing you need to know about saturated fats is they are solid at room temperature, like cheese, milk, butter, poultry skin, and certain other animal meats containing fats. Then there are liquid oils called trans fats, which are turned into solid fat. These are usually found in processed foods. These should be totally eliminated if possible and replaced with good fats such as the monosaturated or polysaturated fats (olive oil, canola oil, soybean oil, nuts, and peanut butter).

Remember, it is important to have some fats in your diet, but try to replace the bad fats with the good fats to help reduce your risks of any complications of "da suga."

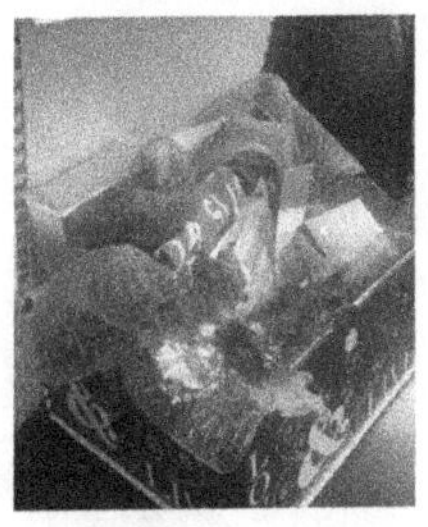

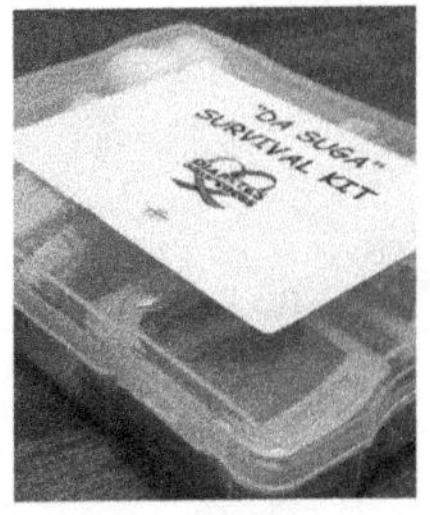

"DA SUGA" SURVIVAL KIT

"Da Suga" Survival Kit is just that. It contains all of the items necessary to check blood sugar levels and provide treatment. Since so many people have diabetes, there should be a survival kit in every first-aid station, church, airport, or any other place where people congregate.

Remember, although there is no cure for diabetes, it is a disease that can be managed through diet and exercise. Know your family history so that you may be able to safeguard yourself from developing this disease.

"Love a prick, save a limb.
Check 'da suga' often!"

TRUSTED RESOURCES

Ignatavicius, D.D, Workman, M.R. (2010). Medical Surgical Nursing and Patient Centered Collaborative Care (6th ed.) St. Louis, MO, Saunders Elsevier.

Jaret, P. (2014, October) Eight Facts About Diabetes That Could Save Your Life. AARP Bulletin/Real Possibilities pp. 10-12.

Diabetes Basics. (n.d.). Retrieved September 9, 2014, from http://www.diabetes.org/diabetes-basics/

American Diabetes Association. (n.d.). Retrieved June 15, 2014, from http://www.diabetes.org/

Diabetes Care. (n.d.). Retrieved October 11, 2014, from http://care.diabetesjournals.org/

Hortensius, RN, J., Slingerland, PHD, R., Kleefstra, MD, PHD, N., Log-tenberg, MD, PHD, S., Groenier, PHD, K., Houweling, MD, PHD, S., & Bi-lo, MD, PHD, H. (n.d.). Self-Monitoring of Blood Glucose: The Use of the First of the Second Drop of Blood. Retrieved October 11, 2014, from http://care.diabetesjournals.org/content/early/2011/02/01/d10-1694

Rotating Your Injection Sites. (n.d.). Retrieved October 9, 2014, from http://www.bd.com/us/diabetes/page.aspx?cat=7001&id=7282

MORE TRUSTED RESOURCES

WebMD Common Health Topics A-Z

Find reliable health and medical information on common topics from A to Z. (n.d.). Retrieved December 16, 2014, from http://www.webmd.com/a-to-z-guides/common-topics/default.htm

WebMD—Better information

Better health. (n.d.). Retrieved November 9, 2014, from http://www.webmd.com/

www.ingramcontent.com/pod-product-compliance
Lightning Source LLC
Chambersburg PA
CBHW060741280326
41934CB00010B/2302

* 9 7 8 1 9 4 3 2 5 8 7 8 9 *